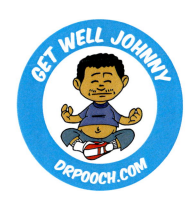

GET WELL JOHNNY
Book 1: Sugar From Nature Is Always Fine!

By Dr. Pooch

Illustrations by Cuzzin' Dave

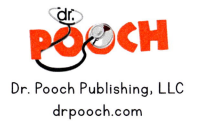

Dr. Pooch Publishing, LLC
drpooch.com

Get Well Johnny
Book 1: Sugar From Nature Is Always Fine!
Copyright © 2015 by Dr. Pooch
Published by Dr. Pooch Publishing, LLC

ALL RIGHTS RESERVED. No part of this book shall be reproduced without written consent from the publisher, except for brief excerpts for the purpose of review.

ISBN: 978-0-9964667-2-1

DISCLAIMER: Dr. Pooch is NOT a medical doctor. Therefore, the information within this book is for educational purposes only. It should not be used as a substitute for professional medical advice, diagnosis or treatment regarding your or your child's well-being.

For more info: visit drpooch.com

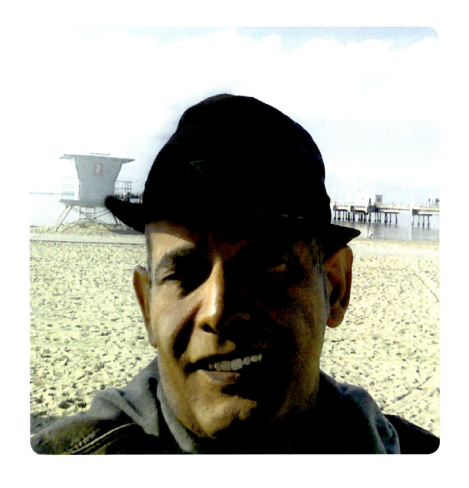

This book is dedicated to Dave "Cuzzin' Dave" Rodriguez, who lost his battle with cancer during the making of this book series. He was a one-of-a-kind guy with a great sense of humanity and humor.

Before the "Get Well Johnny" series, Cuzzin' Dave worked on Charlie Brown, Teenage Mutant Ninja Turtles and more. May his memory be honored by any who've gained insight from the wisdom within this book.

May you rest in peace, Cuzzin' Dave.

NOTE TO PARENTS

Sugar in its refined form (and refined products in general) is one of the leading causes of mineral deficiencies and, furthermore, disease in our country. With dozens of adverse effects, one may think that such a product would come with warning labels indicating its potential hazards or at least not be marketed in products so indiscriminately to our children as a healthy substitute for natural food and water.

Refined sugar has an incredible addiction-forming ability. This fact has been widely known and well-documented throughout the global scientific community for many years, yet seldom discussed in popular culture. Refinement simply means the separation of all minerals (life elements) present in a whole natural food. Thus, when ingested, the body must deplete its own mineral content to process/digest this food-like substance.

So, feeding refined products to your child (or consuming them yourself) literally means you are depleting their/your mineral content, especially if not balancing these manufactured "foods" with Whole Organic Natural Food. The over-consumption of refined sugars in drinks and food is the leading cause of Diabetes, Cancer, Obesity, ADHD, Insomnia, Constipation, Acne, Asthma, Tooth Decay, Eczema, Arthritis and other chronic illnesses and diseases.
-Dr. Pooch

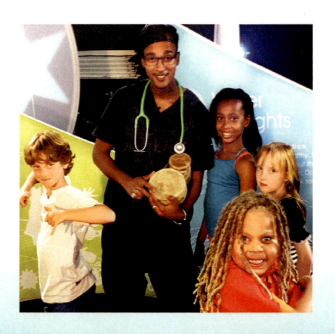

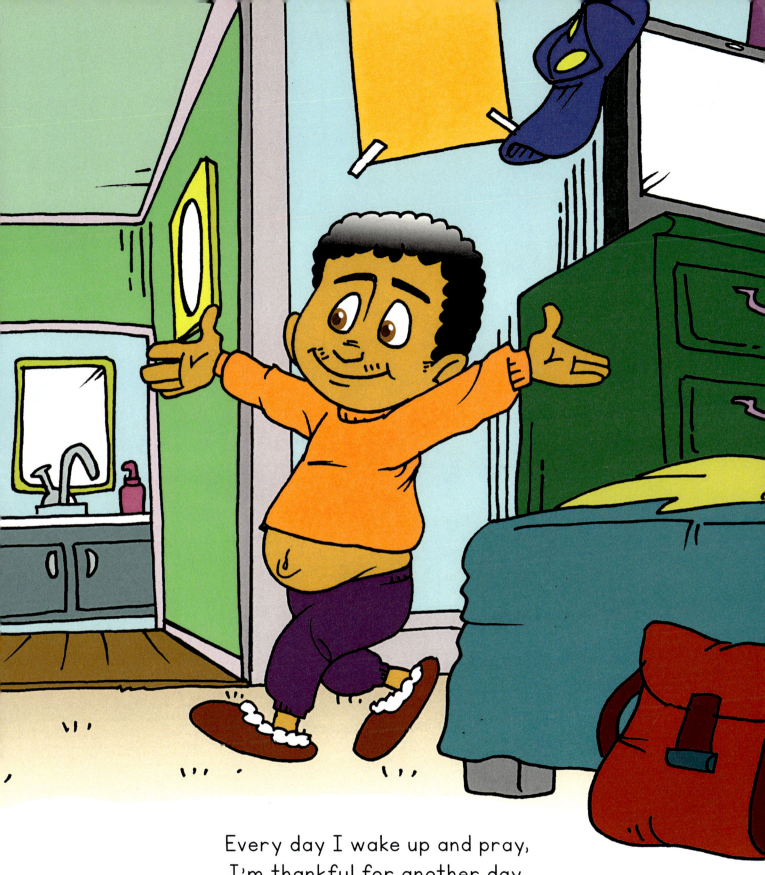

Every day I wake up and pray,
I'm thankful for another day.
I wash my body, then brush my teeth,
and make sure my bed is nice and neat.

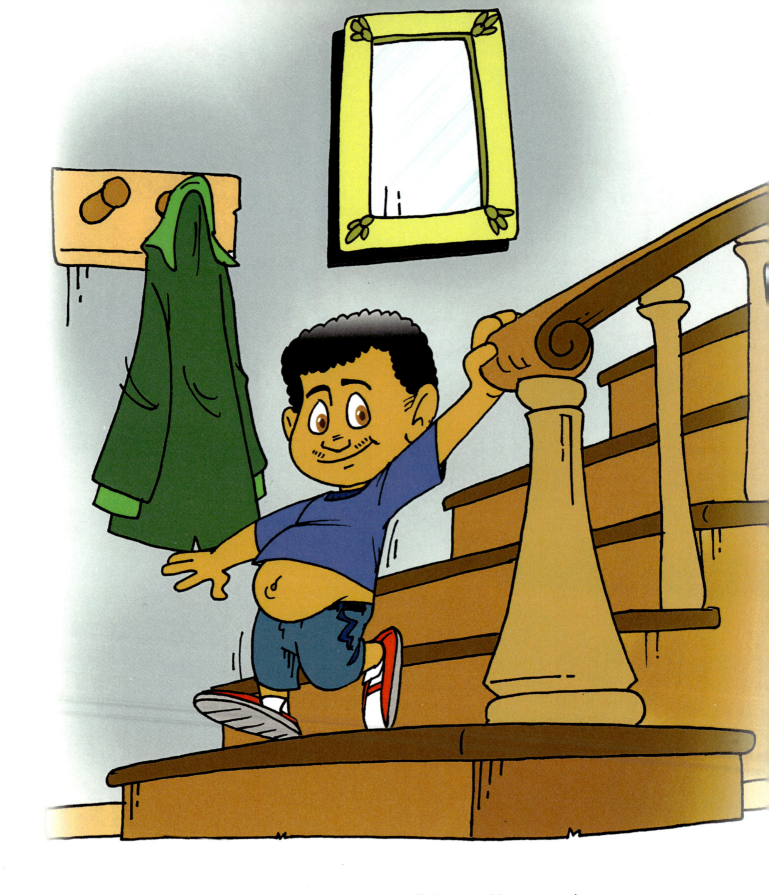

I go downstairs when I hear the words, "Johnny Mustache, breakfast is served."

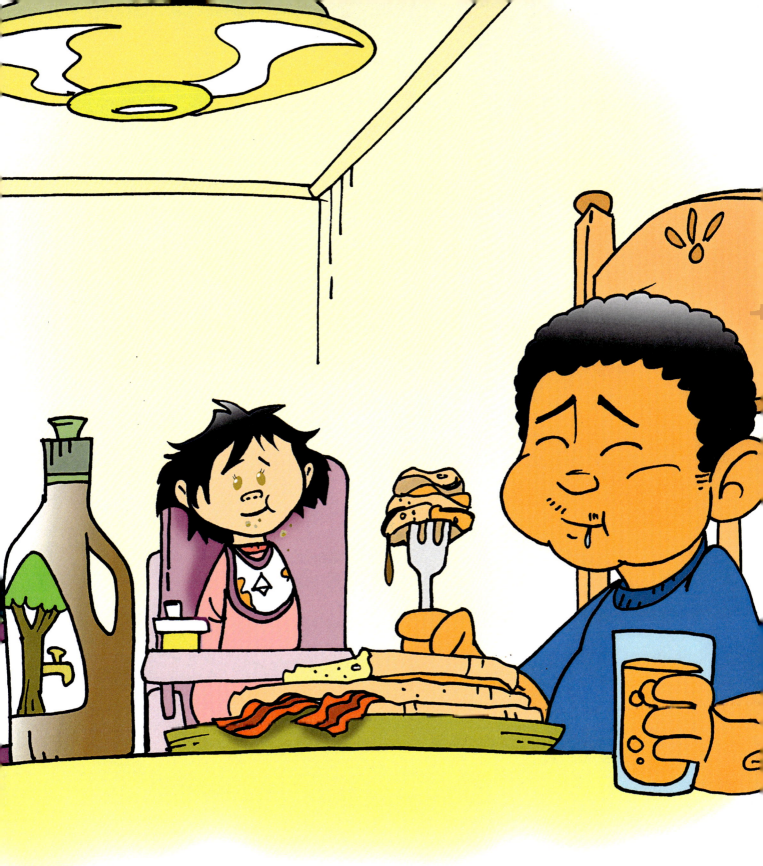

Pancakes with butter, syrup or jelly.
Bacon and eggs all fill my belly.

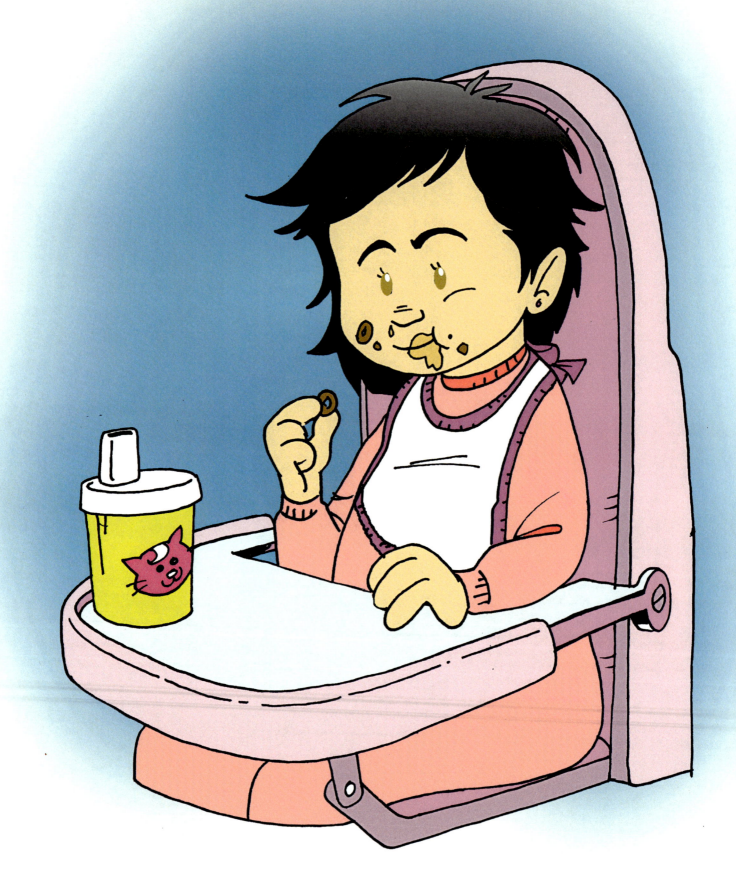

My sister is sick and eats only a little.
Her nose is so runny 'cause she has the sniffles.

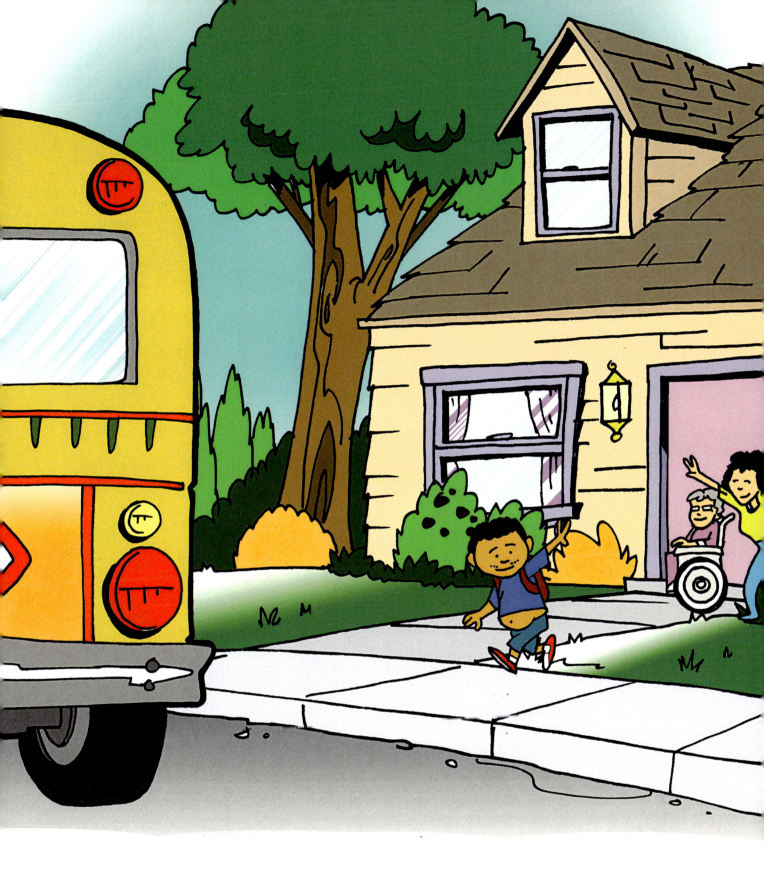

Abuela looks out the window and sees the school bus.
Mommy gives me a kiss and hands me my lunch.

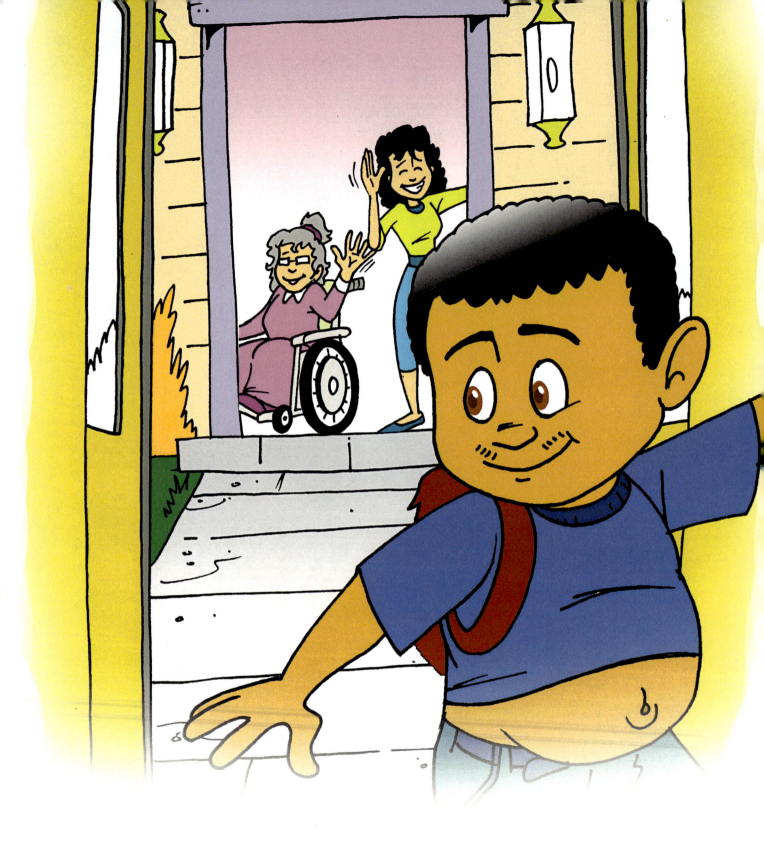

Mom yells, "Dot all your I's and keep your T's crossed!"

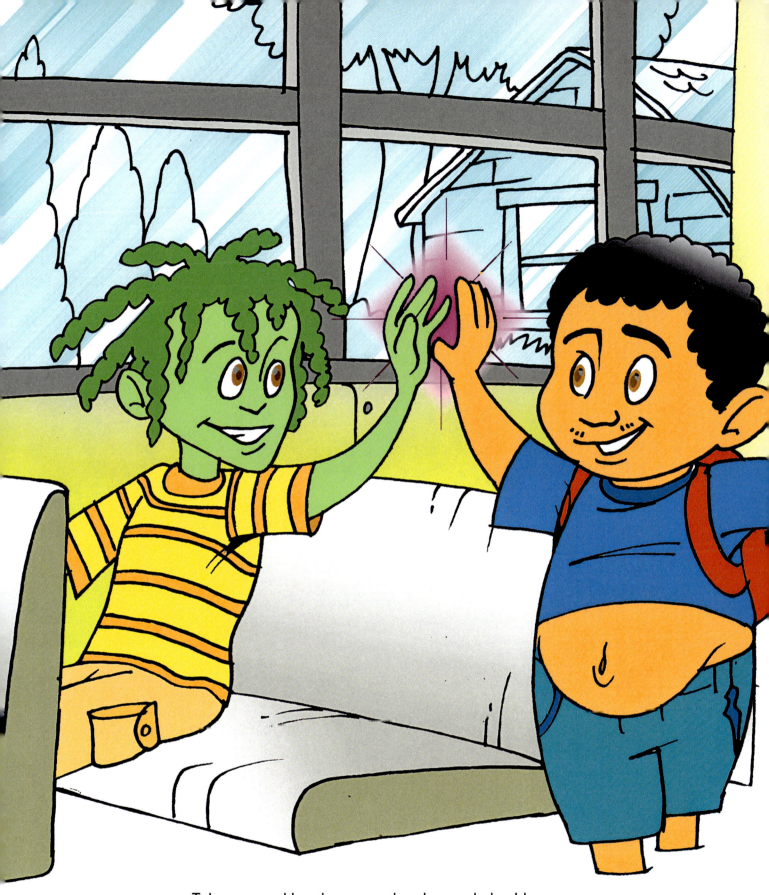

I hop on the bus and sit next to Haas.
Haas Vegetable's my buddy; he and I are a team.

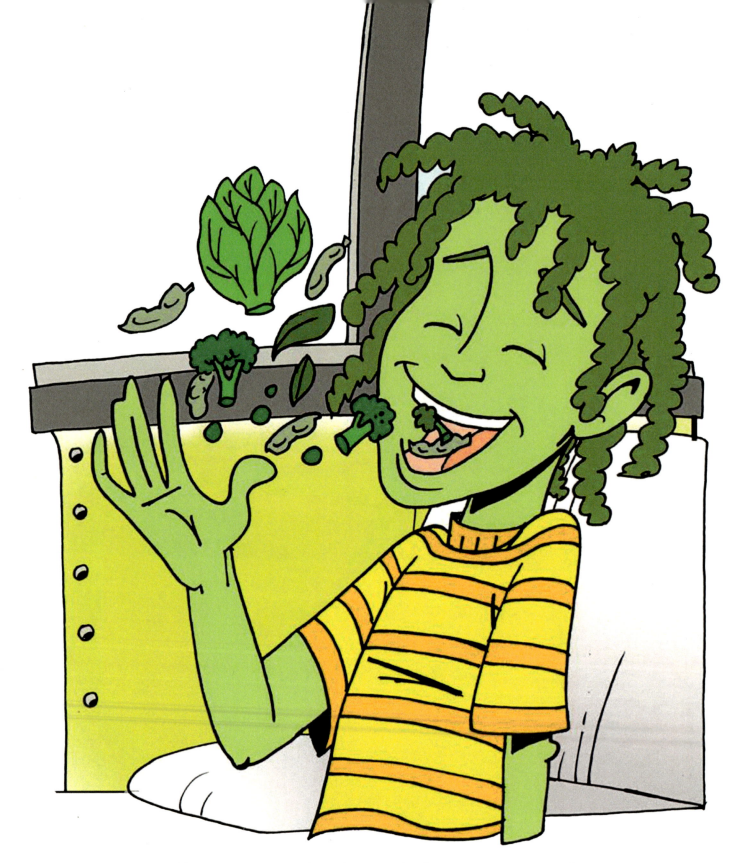

His hair is so bushy and skin is so green!
He eats foods like kale and broccoli stems,
or spinach and peas. He's such a good friend.

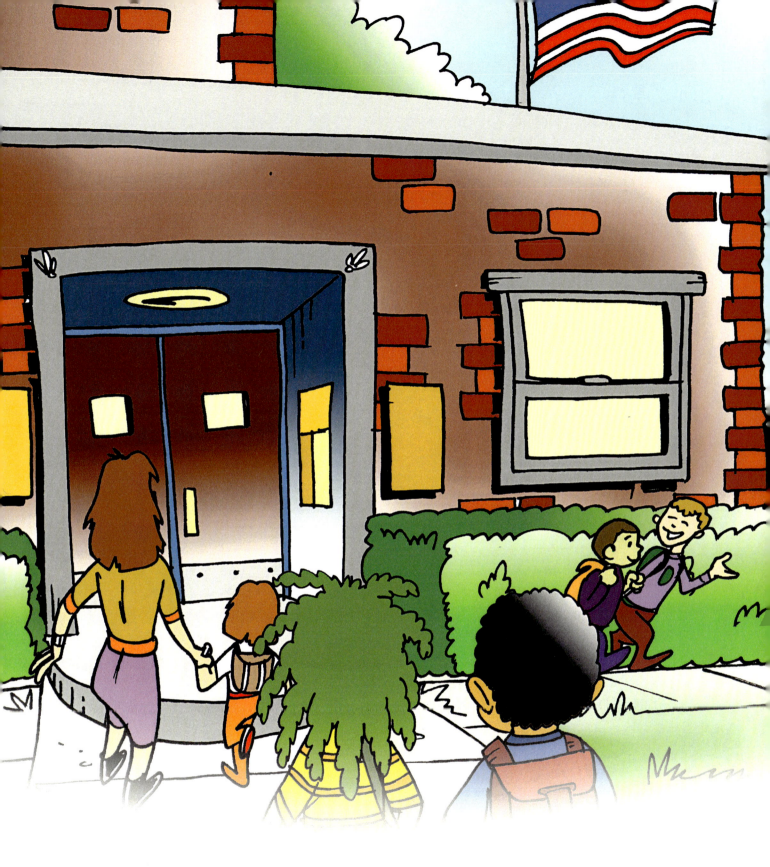

"Hooray!" I say. "We've made it to school.
I wonder, today, what we'll learn that's cool?!"

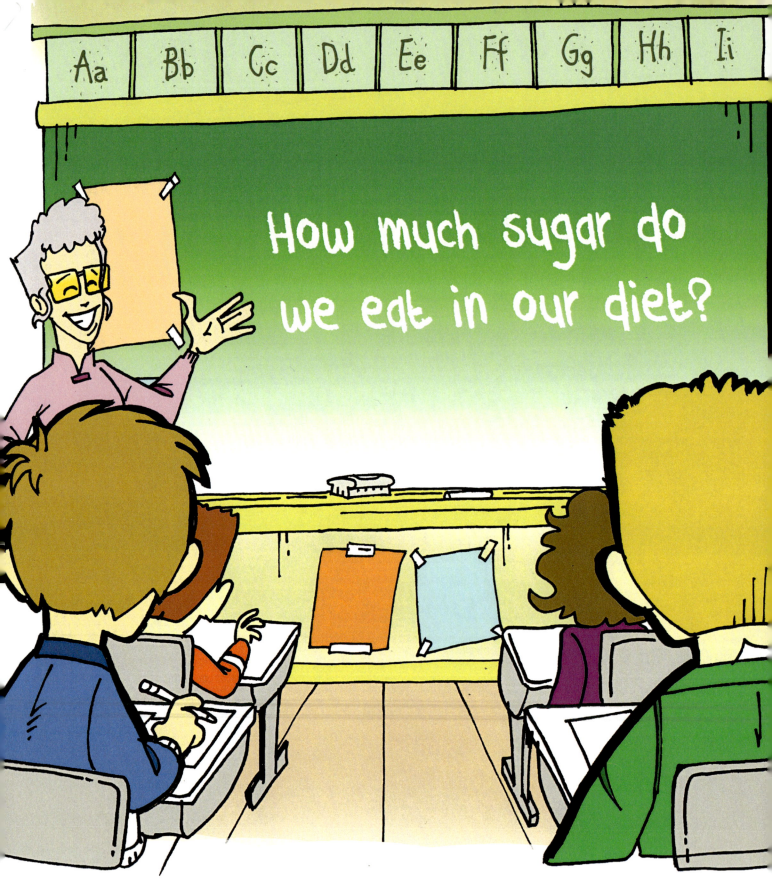

Mrs. Facts said in class, "Today, we're learning the science of how much sugar we eat in our diets."

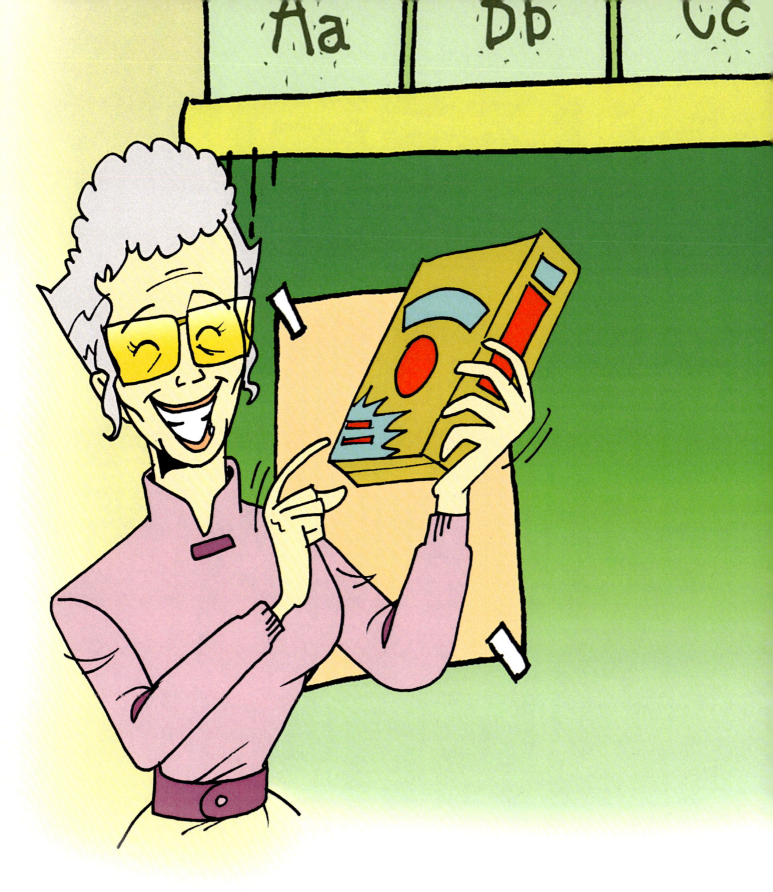

She taught us, "Before food reaches the table…"

Nutrition Facts

Serving Size 1
Servings Per Container 1

Amount Per Serving

Calories 300   Calories From Fat 45

% Daily Value

Total Fat 5g	8%
Saturated Fat 1.5g	8%
Trans Fat 0g	
Cholesterol 30mg	10%
Sodium 430mg	18%
Total Carbohydrate 55g	18%
Dietary Fiber 6g	24%
Sugars 23g	
Protein 14g	

Vitamin A 15%   Vitamin C 0%
Calcium 4%   Iron 2%

*Percent Daily Values are based on a 2,000 calorie diet. Your Daily Values may be higher or lower depending on your calorie needs:

		2,000	2,500
	Calories:		
Total Fat	Less than	65g	80g
Saturated Fat	Less than	20g	25g
Cholesterol	Less than	300mg	300mg
Sodium	Less than	2,400mg	2,400mg
Total Carbohydrate		300g	375g
Dietary Fiber		25g	30g

Ingredients: HIGH FRUCTOSE CORN SYRUP, SUGAR, SALT, VEGETABLE OIL, MODIFIED POTATO STARCH, NATURAL AND ARTIFICIAL FLAVOR, ARTIFICIAL COLOR (YELLOW 5, BLUE 1), POTASSIUM SORBATE (PRESERVATIVE).

"Make sure you read the ingredients labels!".

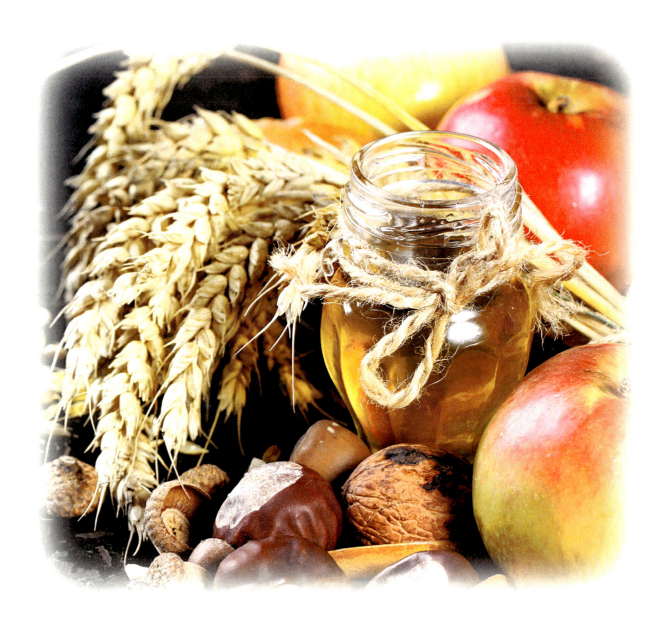

She said, "Sugar from nature is always fine."

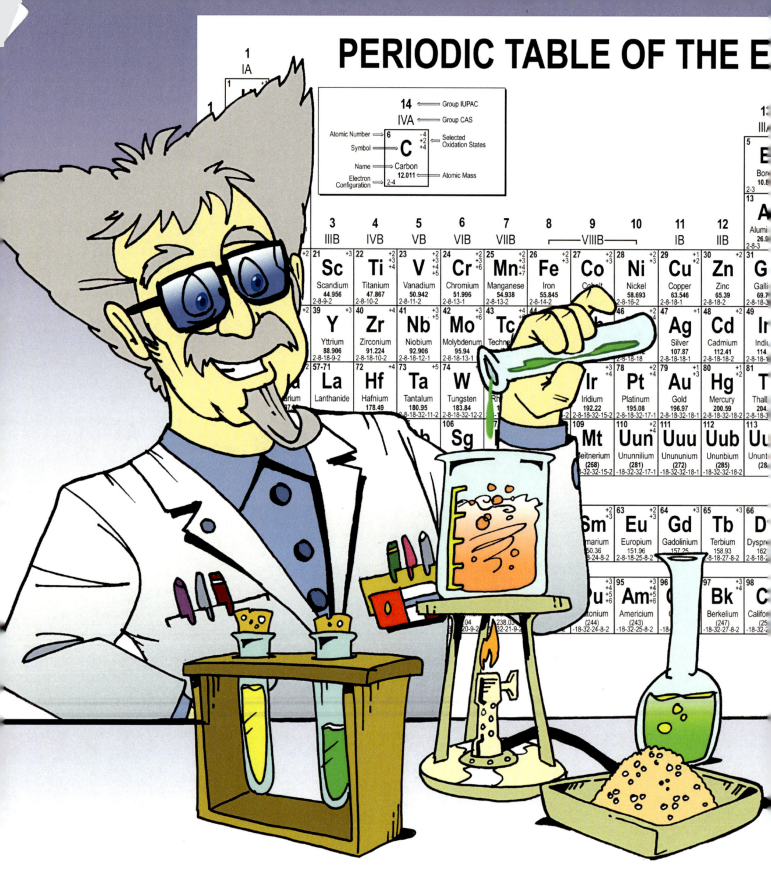

"It's only a hazard when sugar's refined!"

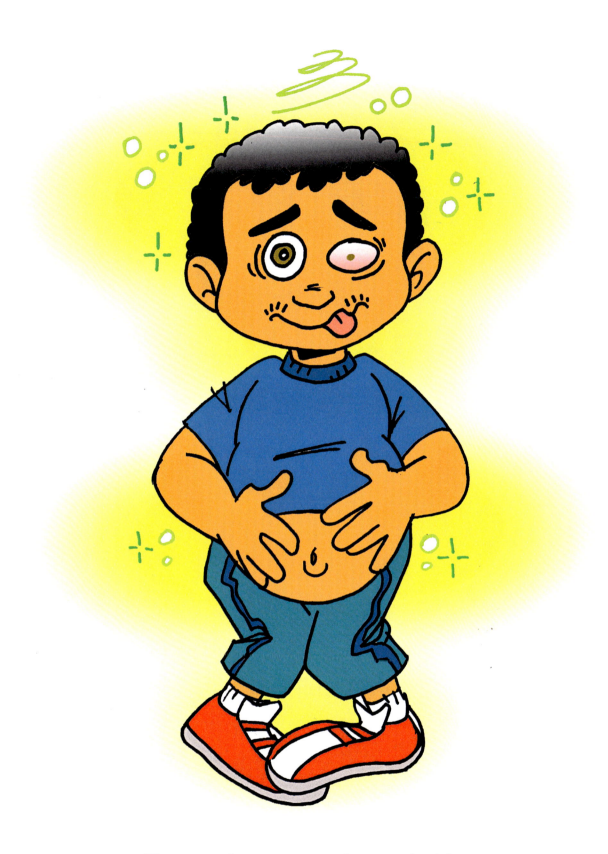

"Too much sugar is always to blame
whenever you're sick and your body's in pain!"

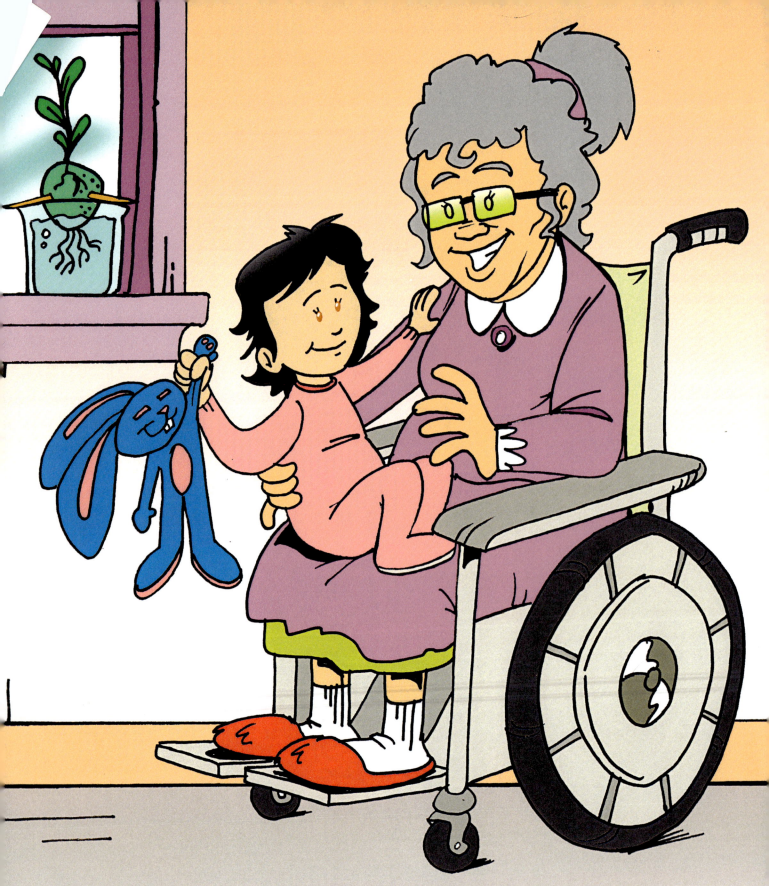

I'm so excited about all that I've learned,
I can't wait to help my sister and Abuela in turn!

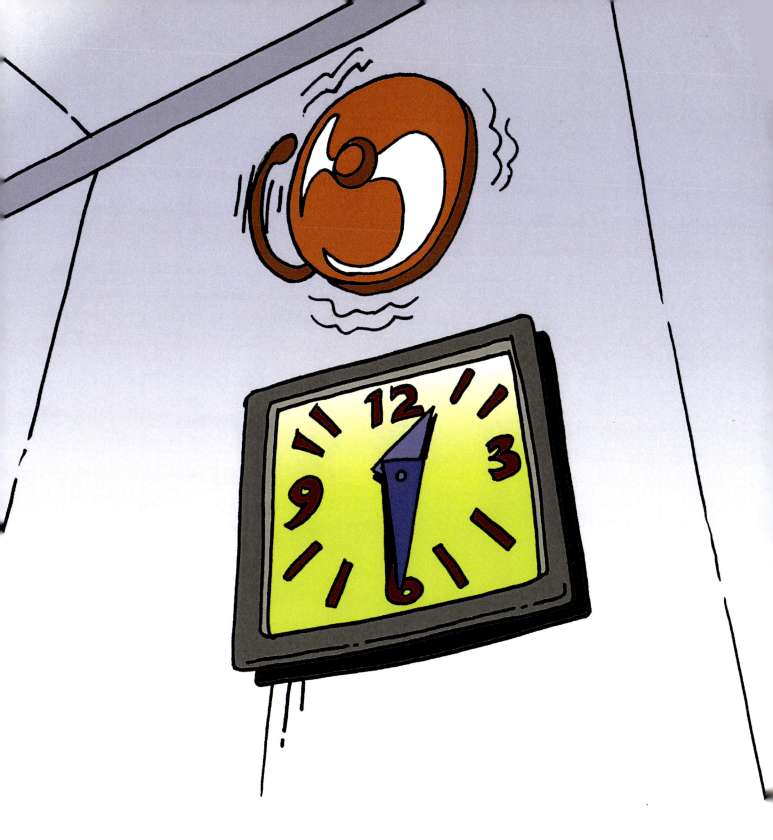

IT'S LUNCHTIME!

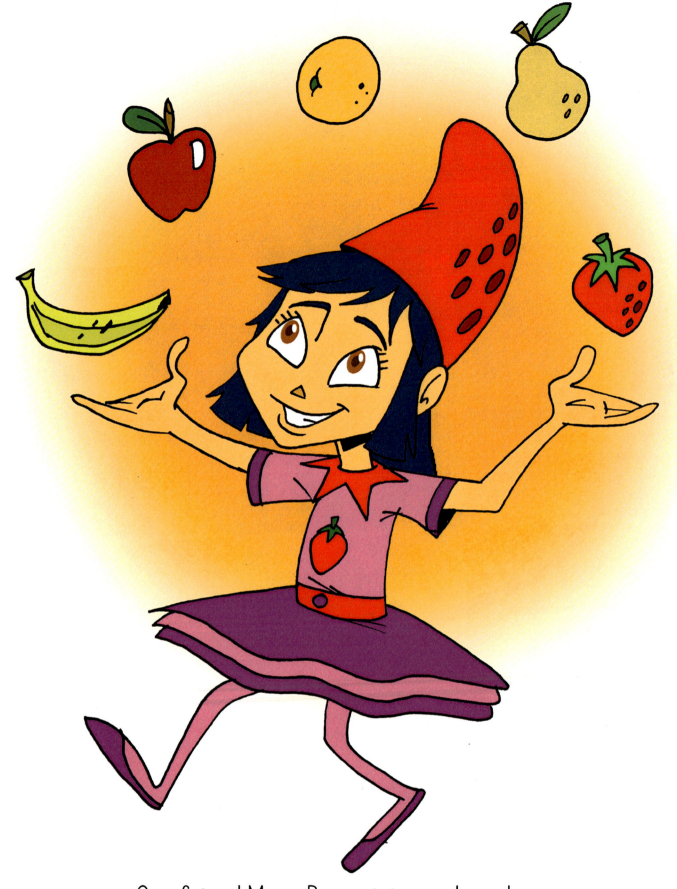

Our friend Mary Berry joins us to eat
with all types of berries, a banana and peach.

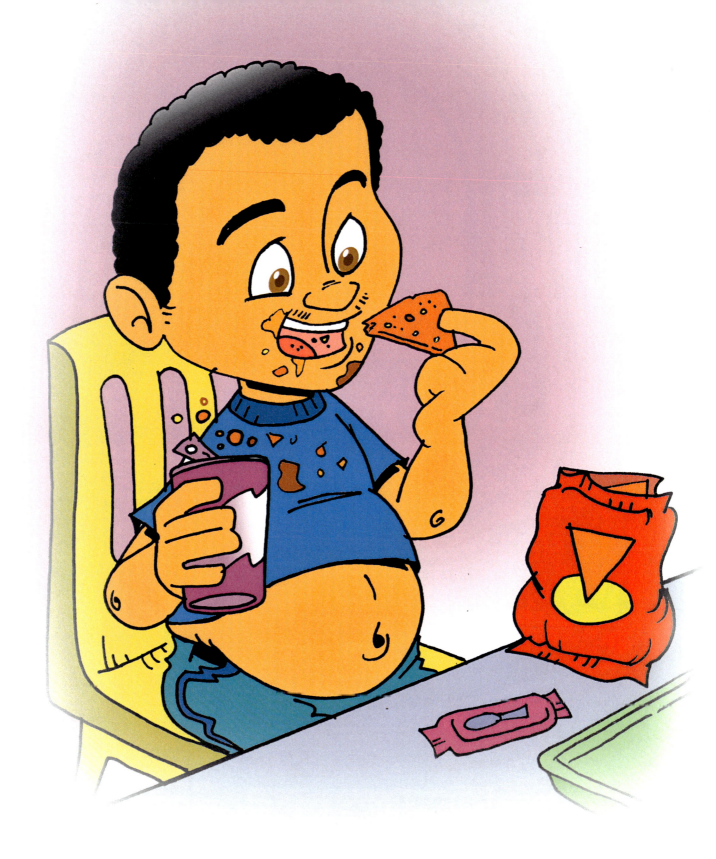

"What are you eating, Mustache!?"
Mrs. Facts told the students,
"Don't eat junk food if you're wise and prudent."

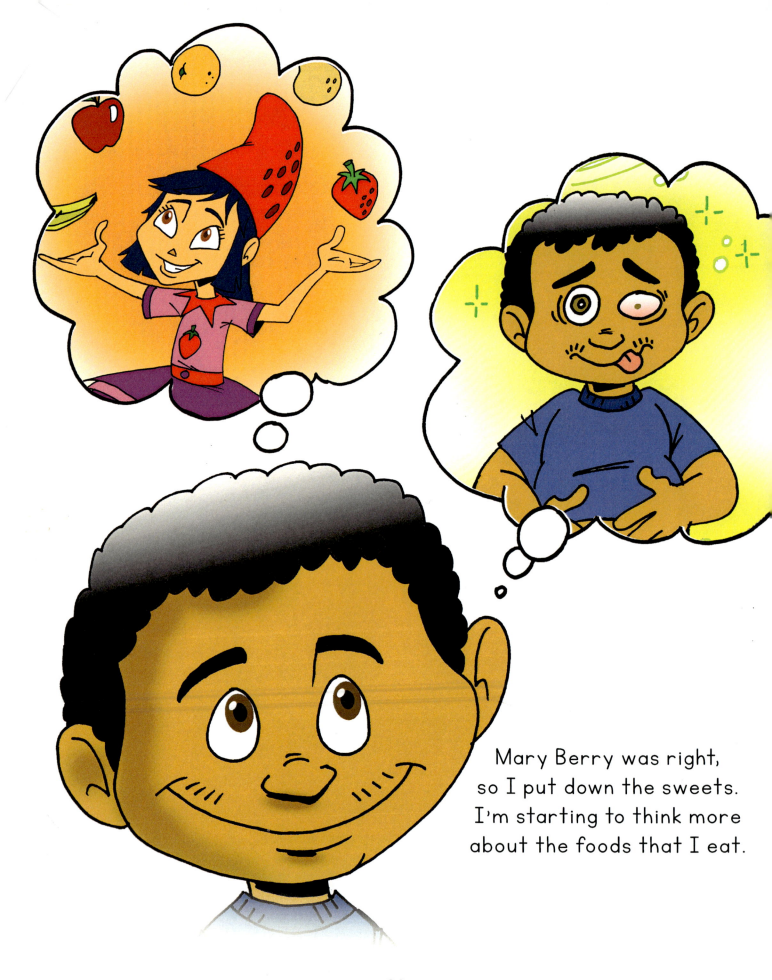

Mary Berry was right, so I put down the sweets. I'm starting to think more about the foods that I eat.

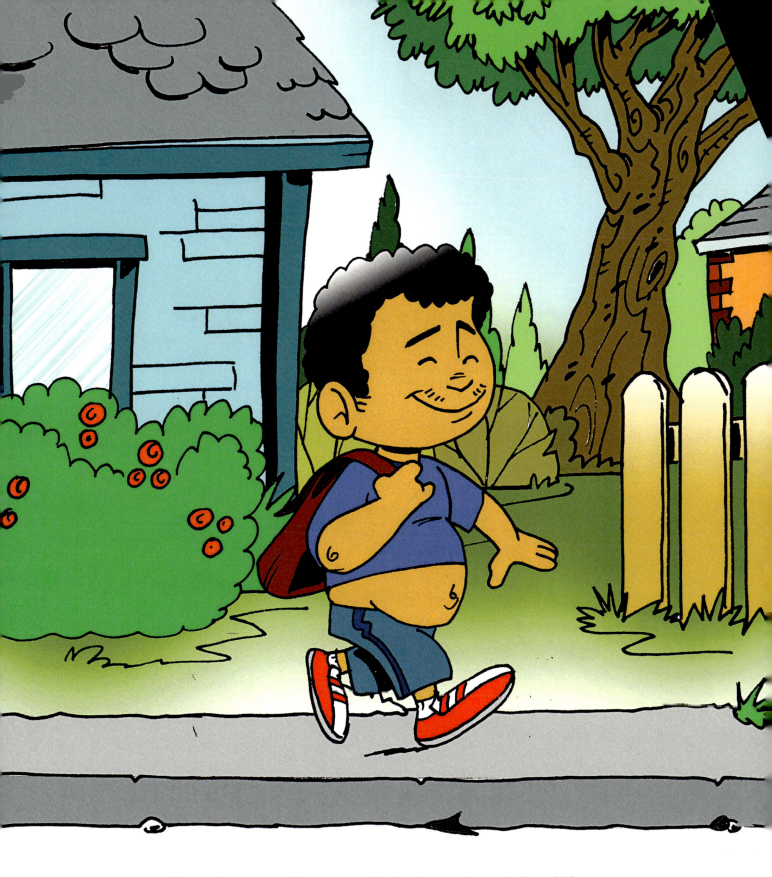

I've learned so much today about health.
I can't wait to go home to my family and help.

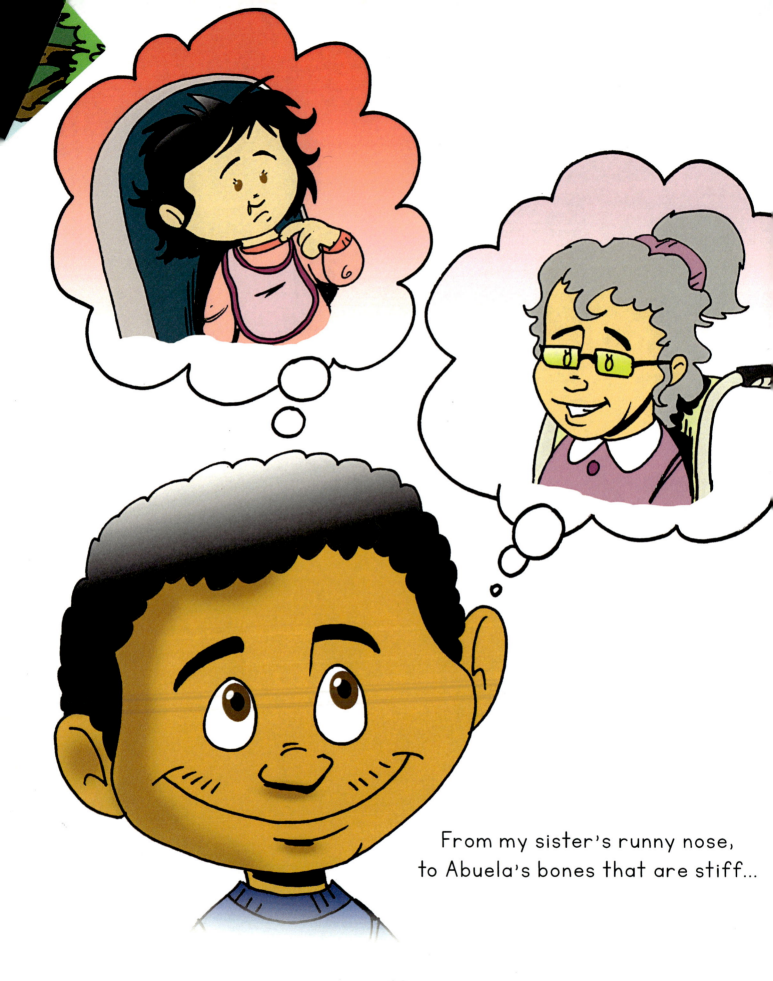

From my sister's runny nose, to Abuela's bones that are stiff...

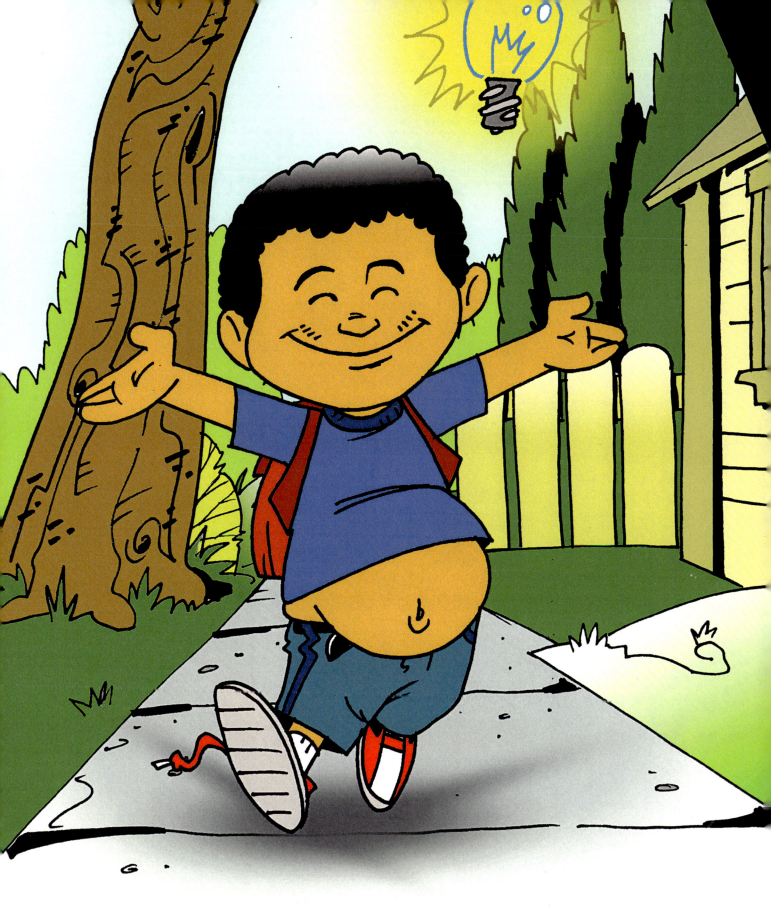

Too much sugar may be the cause of all of it!

Mommy asked what I learned at school. I said, "A lot! We learned which sugars are good and which ones are not!"

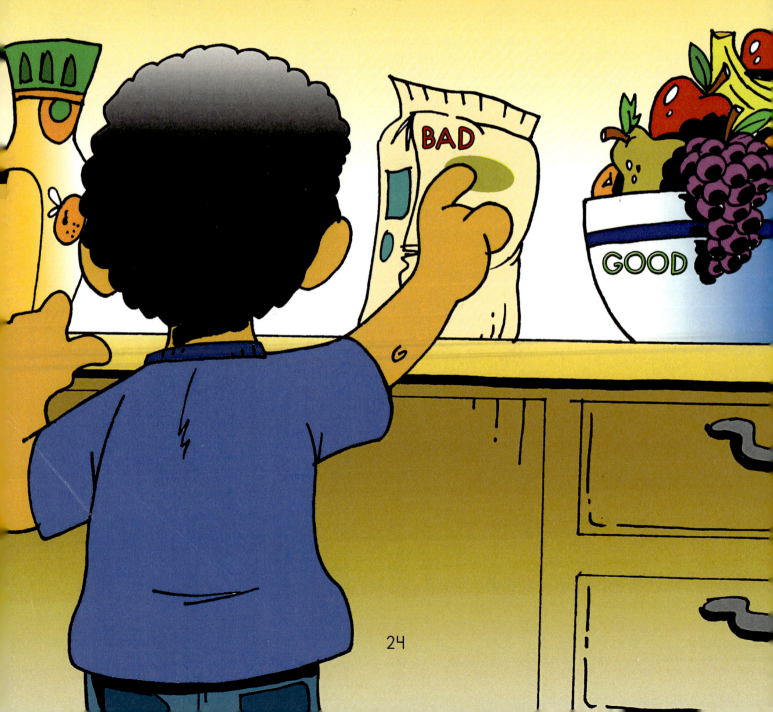

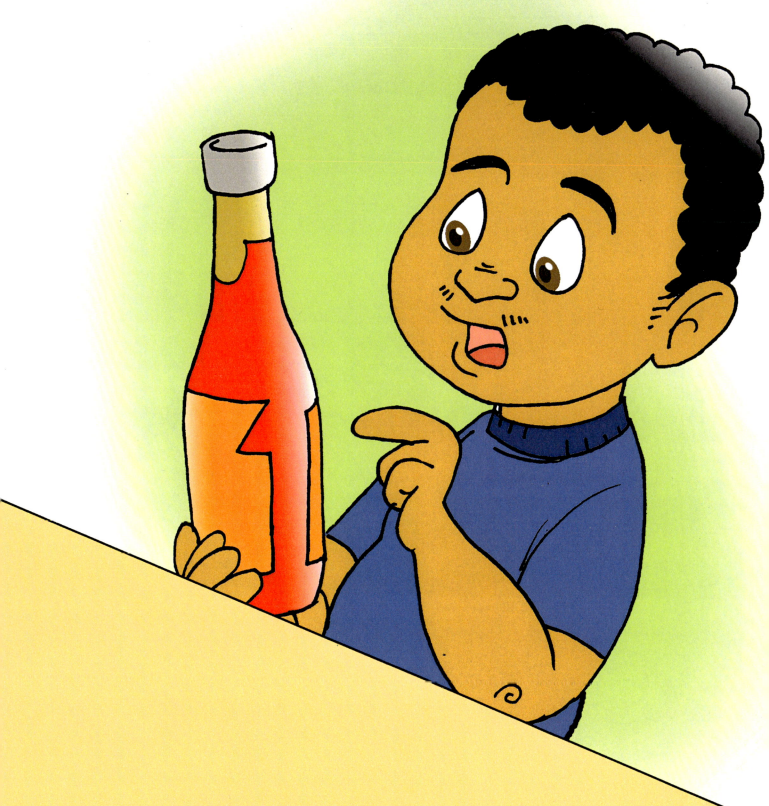

We learned that sugar is hidden under many disguises,
but reading the label is where you will find it.
We learned that sugar has many different names.
Like high fructose corn syrup or sugar cane.

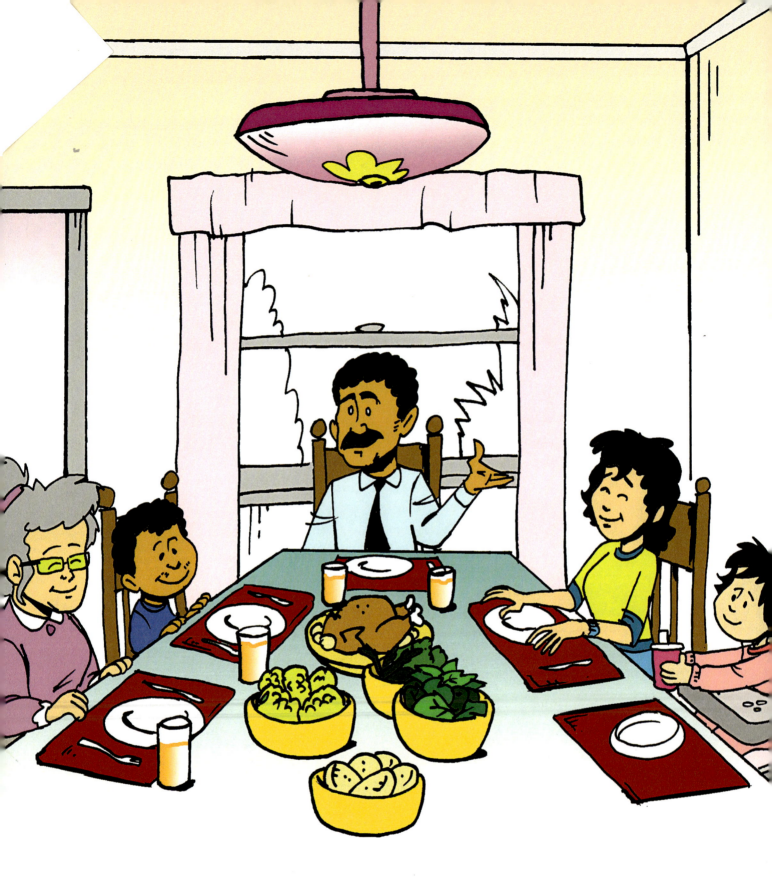

So tonight, for dinner, instead of drive-thru deals...
Let's eat at home and have a wholesome meal.

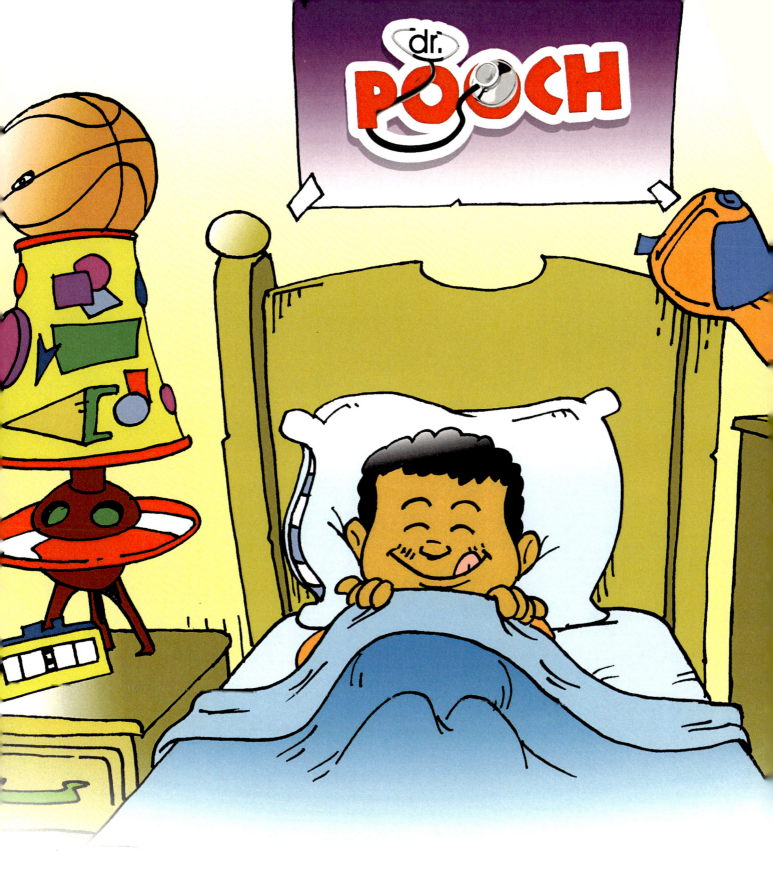

And before bedtime, instead of praying for myself, from now on I'll pray for my family's health."

Fresh Homemade Almond Milk

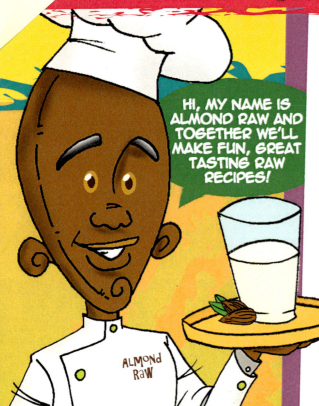

Hi, my name is Almond Raw and together we'll make fun, great tasting raw recipes!

What You'll Need Is:
- 1 Cup Soaked Raw Almonds
- 2 Cups Spring Water
- Agave or Honey To Taste (optional)
- 1 Teaspoon 100% Pure Vanilla Extract (Alcohol Free Preferred) (optional)
- 1 Pinch of Cinnamon (optional)
- 1 Pinch of Nutmeg (optional)
- 1 Teaspoon of Organic Cacao Powder (optional)
- Blender
- 1 Gallon Pitcher (for storage)
- 1 Cheese Cloth (to strain the pulp)

Instructions:
1. Soak almonds in water for up to 24 hours (if time does not permit, for at least 5 minutes).
2. Strain the water from the soaked almonds and place in blender. Dispose of the water.
3. Grind the almonds as finely as possible.
4. Add 1 tablespoon of vanilla extract, 2 tablespoons of agave extract (or honey), cinnamon and nutmeg, and continue blending for another 2 minutes.
5. Strain blended almond milk with cheese cloth to separate the almond pulp from the milk. You may have to repeat a few times to get the milk consistency you wish.
6. Milk is best served chilled. Enjoy!

Almond Banana Ice Cream

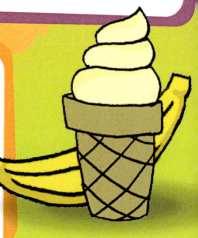

Another Cool Idea:
You can use the almond pulp you strained from your almond milk. The night before you make the almond milk, slice 5 bananas in chunks and freeze them overnight. The next day, when you get ready to make some fresh milk, take the frozen bananas out and rinse them with water. Let them slightly thaw while you make the milk. Mix the remaining almond pulp into the blender along with the frozen bananas. Blend for 2 minutes; pour in a 1/2 Cup of almond milk to the mix; use discretion for desired thickness. Now you have fresh banana almond soft serve ice cream!

READ THE LABEL!
ALWAYS READ THE NUTRITION FACTS

SOME OF SUGAR'S DISGUISES

HIGH FRUCTOSE CORN SYRUP
CORNSTARCH · MALTODEXTRIN
ARTIFICIAL FLAVORS · MALTOSE
DEXTROSE · FRUIT JUICE CONCENTRATE
SORBITOL · CARAMEL COLOR

Refined sugar hides under many disguises. Each one of the names listed above is either a refined, processed and/or synthetic form of sugar. The human body does not recognize these as nutrition. Our body does not know how to properly digest and use these fake sugars as fuel (energy). Instead, the body will store them as fat, acid and/or inflammation.

Nutrition Facts

Serving Size 1
Servings Per Container 1

Amount Per Serving

Calories 300 | Calories From Fat 45

	% Daily Value
Total Fat 5g	
Saturated Fat 1.5g	8%
Trans Fat 0g	8%
Cholesterol 30mg	
Sodium 430mg	10%
Total Carbohydrate 55g	18%
Dietary Fiber 6g	18%
Sugars 23g	24%
Protein 14g	

Vitamin A 15%   Vitamin C 0%
Calcium 4%   Iron 2%

*Percent Daily Values are based on a 2,000 calorie diet. Your Daily Values may be higher or lower depending on your calorie needs:

	Calories:	2,000	2,500
Total Fat	Less than	65g	80g
Saturated Fat	Less than	20g	25g
Cholesterol	Less than	300mg	300mg
Sodium	Less than	2,400mg	2,400mg
Total Carbohydrate		300g	375g
Dietary Fiber		25g	30g

Ingredients: HIGH FRUCTOSE CORN SYRUP, SUGAR, SALT, VEGETABLE OIL, MODIFIED POTATO STARCH, NATURAL AND ARTIFICIAL FLAVOR, ARTIFICIAL COLOR (YELLOW 5, BLUE 1), POTASSIUM SORBATE (PRESERVATIVE).

> REMEMBER:
> "SUGAR FROM NATURE IS ALWAYS FINE; IT'S ONLY A HAZARD WHEN SUGAR'S REFINED."

FIND THE REFINED SUGARS!

AT HOME FIND A SUGARY FOOD INGREDIENT LABEL AND WRITE THE NAME OF AT LEAST 2 REFINED SUGARS BELOW.

_____
_____

NATURAL SUGAR

CIRCLE THE FOODS THAT CONTAIN NATURAL SUGAR!

1. 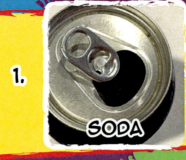 SODA OR 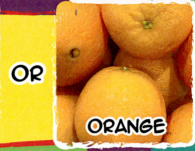 ORANGE

2. 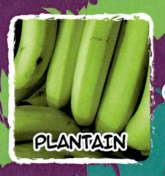 PLANTAIN OR 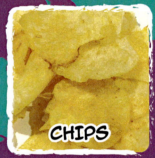 CHIPS

3. 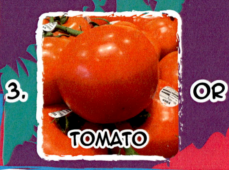 TOMATO OR 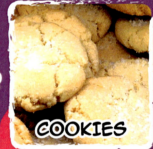 COOKIES

HANG MAN

WHAT IS HARMFUL TO YOUR HEALTH AND IN ALL JUNK FOODS?

_ _ _ _ _ E _

S _ _ _ _

KEY: CIRCLE THE FOOD: 1. ORANGE 2. PLANTAIN 3. TOMATO
HANGMAN: REFINED SUGAR

Sugar from Nature is Always Fine!

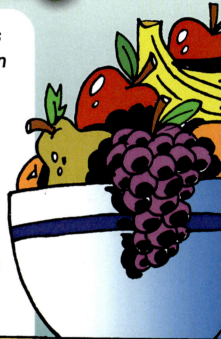

Learning to properly identify natural and refined sugars could mean the difference between health and illness in years to come. In today's modern food markets it is essential to teach our new generation of consumers to properly read and identify harmful ingredients on labels. This early age children's book is a great tool to motivate young minds to seek healthy lives. The Get Well Johnny Book Series is a must have for families and educators looking to initiate young minds into the world of health and wellness! This story is reinforced by exercises and a recipe to engage children and adults.

THANK YOU FOR YOUR DEDICATION TO A HEALTHY FUTURE!

Follow Johnny Mustache in his other adventures!

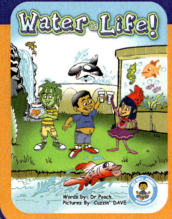
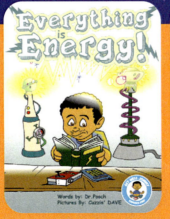
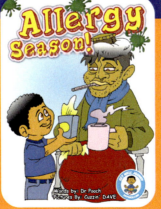
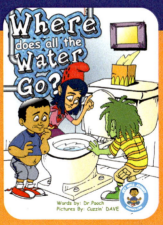

For more info and to purchase your own set of Get Well Johnny books, visit us at: drpooch.com

Made in the USA
Middletown, DE
26 January 2017